THE LAYER SYSTEM

Your Ultimate Skin Care Regime

To Flawless Skin

By Ori Laor

Disclaimer

The information contained within this eBook is strictly for educational purposes. If you wish to apply ideas contained in this eBook, you are taking full responsibility for your actions.

The author has made every effort to ensure the accuracy of the information within this book was correct at time of publication. The author does not assume and at this moment disclaims any liability to any party for any loss, damage, or disruption caused by errors or omissions, whether such errors or omissions result from accident, negligence, or any other cause.

Thank you very much
Ori Laor

Table of Contents

Personal Introduction

Thank you for downloading this fantastic guide - **"THE LAYER SYSTEM - Your Ultimate Skin Care Regime To Flawless Skin"** this book will teach you the secret of young looking skin in any age. The Layer System gives the best answer for Anti-aging, wrinkles and pigmentation and it is keeping the skin alive and glamourous all at the comfort of your home.

Skin is the body's largest organ. It is also the most visible. A square inch of skin has millions of cells and many nerve endings for sensing temperature, pain, pressure, and touch. It keeps us sheltered from the elements and protects our insides from drying up. Yet despite its toughness, skin is sensitive and can be damaged if it isn't cared for. It requires our protection from the sun and from irritants. It needs our help in retaining moisture. It demands a little thought now and then.

Everyone is looking for the fountain of youth, the layer system is definitely one of this fountains. For More than three decades I see results of treatments with the layer system on thousands of people.

Aging is inevitable. Looking your age doesn't have to be! By picking up this book, you've taken the first step to turning back the clock and protecting your skin from future damage and aging. Whether you've already seen the major signs of skin aging (like crow's feet, age spots, dulled complexion, fine lines and wrinkles) or you're eager to delay them as long as possible, you'll find great anti- aging tips and tricks here that you can put to work today!

Today, the battle against aging means that women are fighting against much more than just wrinkles. This handbook will take you step-by-step through the various challenges your skin faces: everything from stress to pollution to weather to proper nutrition, presenting advice and solutions at every step along the way. You'll also get a deeper understanding of how your skin is changing at each stage in your life.

Biological changes may happen like clockwork, but by understanding the changes, you can best target their root causes so the results never show up on your face! It's time to look as young as you feel. Your age can remain your little secret!

Combining scientific research with practical tips that anyone can follow, The Anti-Aging Handbook is your new source for everything anti-aging. The mystical fountain of youth hasn't been found just yet, but the advice and information you'll find in this book is the next best thing!

In this book, you will learn all about your skin and how to take care of it with layer system. You will learn about natural skincare product, and there benefits. Finally, we will look at the seven layers of the skin and how to take care of them.

The Skin-Aging Process

Your skin changes constantly throughout our lives. These changes are as not only relentless, but also diverse. With impacts ranging from wrinkling to discoloration, sagging, redness, age spots, and more, the sooner you can begin your battle against all of the visible signs of aging, the better!

Luckily, these changes to our skin don't happen all at once or suddenly appear one morning when we look in the mirror! Instead, they are more gradual.

Importantly, certain changes are more likely to show up at particular times in our lives because of the specific ways that skin aging occurs during the lifespan.

Recognizing when each change will begin occurring or escalate in intensity can help you to begin taking the necessary preventive and corrective measures when your skin needs them most.

The skin ages in three major ways.

The first is chronological aging. The rate of chronological aging your skin will undergo is influenced by several factors including your genes, hormones, and time. The next section of your handbook will focus on the specific changes over time in the chronological aging process.

The second major way that the skin ages is through photo-aging. Photo- aging is influenced by repeated exposure to UVA and UVB rays, typically from direct, unprotected sun or tanning bed exposure. Preventing and correcting the impact of photo-aging is critical for skin and total body health and will be covered in later chapters.

The third category consists of miscellaneous "lifestyle" factors that can speed up the appearance of aging on your skin. These lifestyle factors include smoking, sleep deprivation, stress, pollution exposure, and more.

In the later chapter, we will discuss the specific ways that our skin changes as we move into new decades in our lives: from the 20s to the 30s to the 40s to the 50s and beyond! Then, you'll learn the appropriate preventive measures and skincare routines that correspond to preventing and correcting these changes at each stage. Armed with this information, you'll be in the best position to maintain consistently healthy, radiant, and youthful-looking skin, no matter which stage you're currently at!

For my new Kindle and Createspace readers, I offer a Free Voucher Gift of 20$. You can find a keyword at the end of this book. Please send it to my mail orilaor@outlook.com, and you will receive a discount for any porches you make for yourself, a member of your family or a friend in LAOR website www.laorcare.com.

About Me

I have a passion for Beauty, Skincare, Anti-aging and well-being methods. In my extensive exploration around the world, I gathered sacred pieces of information that helped me and then other people from all walks of life to look and feel younger. I hold a BA in Art and diplomas for Makeup Artist,

Para Medical Aesthetician, Aromatherapy, Naturopathy, and Nutrition consultant. I am a well-known name in T.V scene and in the cosmetic industry, including treating many celebrities. When I was 30 years old, I quit working for others and founded LAOR, a House of natural Beauty and Professional Skin Care and treatments for the face, Body, and Mind.

Since an early age, I suffered from my skin and was carried away with Skincare research, science and well-being. I worked in beauty and style departments in New York and Tel Aviv, based on my experience I invented a revolutionary practice for treating the skin from within – **The Layer system**, Complied with a line of professional cosmetic products and treatments for the face to treat any skin problem.

Ientered the natural cosmetics world with a unique world-view and with one simple, honest purpose: to create a different kind of cosmetic that is Natural and effective. My desire is that each product would provide each with the essence of beauty, based on effective ingredients.

Now, for the past Two Decades, I am designing the products that Men and women across the world love, helping them to look and feel younger with all the secrets of skin care. When I am not working, I love to design and create, read, write and paint. My quest is to bring more beauty to the world and raise self-awareness.

Let's Get Started!

Chapter 1

The Layer System

What Is The Layer System?

The skin is built from 7 layers but there are three main layers Of skin and there are layers within two of these layers. One of these layers is the epidermis; the epidermis is the top external layer and has five layers within that layer. The next layer is the dermis; the dermis has two layers within its layer. Then there is the last layer this layer is the hypodermis, the hypodermis is mostly fat and it has no layers within it.

The epidermis has five layers within that layer. The first two layers within the epidermis are called the stratum corundum and the next layer is the stratum lucidum, this is only in thick skin like the palms of your hands and the sole of your foot. Another two layers within the epidermis is the stratum gramnulosum and the stratum spiosum. The last layer within the epidermis is the stratum germinativum. These are the layers within the epidermis.

The dermis has two layers within its layer. The first layer in the dermis is the dermal papillary layer. The next layer within the dermis is the dermal reticular layer; this layer is the location of a lot of structures such as the hair follicles and the blood vessels. These are the layers within the dermis.

Scientific Explanation On The Layers Of The Skin

The Epidermis

The epidermis is composed of keratinized, stratified squamous epithelium. It is made of four or five layers of epithelial cells, depending on its location in the body. It does not have any blood vessels within it (i.e., it is avascular). Skin that has four layers of cells is referred to as "thin skin." From deep to superficial, these layers are the stratum basale, stratum spinosum, stratum granulosum, and stratum corneum. Most of the skin can be classified as thin skin. "Thick skin" is found only on the palms of the hands and the soles of the feet. It has a fifth layer, called the stratum lucidum, located between the stratum corneum and the stratum granulosum

1. Stratum Basale

The stratum basale (also called the stratum germinativum) is the deepest epidermal layer and attaches the epidermis to the basal lamina, below which lie the layers of the dermis. The cells in the stratum basale bond to the dermis via intertwining collagen fibers, referred to as the basement membrane. A finger-like projection, or fold, known as the dermal papilla (plural = dermal papillae) is found in the superficial portion of the dermis. Dermal papillae increase the strength of the connection between the epidermis and dermis; the greater the folding, the stronger the connections made.

The stratum basale is a single layer of cells primarily made of basal cells. A basal cell is a cuboidal-shaped stem cell that is a precursor of the keratinocytes of the epidermis. All of the keratinocytes are produced from this single layer of cells, which are constantly going through mitosis to produce new cells. As new cells are formed, the existing cells are pushed superficially away from the stratum basale. Two other cell types are found dispersed among the basal cells in the stratum basale. The first is a Merkel cell, which functions as a receptor and is responsible for stimulating sensory nerves that the brain perceives as touch. These cells are especially abundant on the surfaces of the hands and feet. The second is a melanocyte, a cell that produces the pigment melanin. Melanin gives hair and skin its color, and also helps protect the living cells of the epidermis from ultraviolet (UV) radiation damage.

In a growing fetus, fingerprints form where the cells of the stratum basale meet the papillae of the underlying dermal layer (papillary layer), resulting in the formation of the ridges on your fingers that you recognize as fingerprints. Fingerprints are unique to each individual and are used for forensic analyses because the patterns do not change with the growth and aging processes.

2. Stratum Spinosum

As the name suggests, the stratum spinosum is spiny in appearance due to the protruding cell processes that join the cells via a structure called a desmosome. The desmosomes interlock with each other and strengthen the bond between the cells. It is interesting to note that the "spiny" nature of this layer is an artifact of the staining process. Unstained epidermis samples do not exhibit this characteristic appearance. The stratum spinosum is composed of eight to 10 layers of keratinocytes, formed as a result of cell division in the stratum basale. Interspersed among the keratinocytes of this layer is a type of dendritic cell called the Langerhans cell, which functions as a macrophage by engulfing bacteria, foreign particles, and damaged cells that occur in this layer.

The keratinocytes in the stratum spinosum begin the synthesis of keratin and release a water-repelling glycolipid that helps prevent water loss from the body, making the skin relatively waterproof. As new keratinocytes are produced atop the stratum basale, the keratinocytes of the stratum spinosum are pushed into the stratum granulosum.

3. Stratum Granulosum

The stratum granulosum has a grainy appearance due to further changes to the keratinocytes as they are pushed from the stratum spinosum. The cells (three to five layers deep) become flatter, their cell membranes thicken, and they generate large amounts of the proteins keratin, which is fibrous, and keratohyalin, which accumulates as lamellar granules within the cells. These two proteins make up the bulk of the keratinocyte mass in the stratum granulosum and give the layer its grainy appearance. The nuclei and other cell organelles disintegrate as the cells die, leaving behind the keratin, keratohyalin, and cell membranes that will form the stratum lucidum, the stratum corneum, and the accessory structures of hair and nails.

4. Stratum Lucidum

The stratum lucidum is a smooth, seemingly translucent layer of the epidermis located just above the stratum granulosum and below the stratum corneum. This thin layer of cells is found only in the thick skin of the palms, soles, and digits. The keratinocytes that compose the stratum lucidum are dead and flattened. These cells are densely packed with eleiden, a clear protein rich in lipids, derived from keratohyalin, which gives these cells their transparent (i.e., lucid) appearance and provides a barrier to water.

5. Stratum Corneum

The stratum corneum is the most superficial layer of the epidermis and is the layer exposed to the outside environment. The increased keratinization (also called cornification) of the cells in this layer gives it its name. There are usually 15 to 30 layers of cells in the stratum corneum. This dry, dead layer helps prevent the penetration of microbes and the dehydration of underlying tissues, and provides a mechanical protection against abrasion for the more delicate, underlying layers. Cells in this layer are shed periodically and are replaced by cells pushed up from the stratum granulosum (or stratum lucidum in the case of the palms and soles of feet). The entire layer is replaced during a period of about 4 weeks. Cosmetic procedures, such as microdermabrasion, help remove some of the dry, upper layer and aim to keep the skin looking "fresh" and healthy.

The Dermis

The dermis might be considered the "core" of the integumentary system (derma- = "skin"), as distinct from the epidermis (epi- = "upon" or "over") and hypodermis (hypo- = "below"). It contains blood and lymph vessels, nerves, and other structures, such as hair follicles and sweat glands. The dermis is made of two layers of connective tissue that compose an interconnected mesh of elastin and collagenous fibers, produced by fibroblasts.

6. Papillary Layer

The papillary layer is made of loose, areolar connective tissue, which means the collagen and elastin fibers of this layer form a loose mesh. This superficial layer of the dermis projects into the stratum basale of the epidermis to form finger-like dermal papillae. Within the papillary layer are fibroblasts, a small number of fat cells (adipocytes), and an abundance of small blood vessels. In addition, the papillary layer contains phagocytes, defensive cells that help fight bacteria or other infections that have breached the skin. This layer also contains lymphatic capillaries, nerve fibers, and touch receptors called the Meissner corpuscles.

7. Reticular Layer

Underlying the papillary layer is the much thicker reticular layer, composed of dense, irregular connective tissue. This layer is well vascularized and has a rich sensory and sympathetic nerve supply. The reticular layer appears reticulated (net-like) due to a tight meshwork of fibers. Elastin fibers provide some elasticity to the skin, enabling movement. Collagen fibers provide structure and tensile strength, with strands of collagen extending into both the papillary layer and the hypodermis. In addition, collagen binds water to keep the skin hydrated. Collagen injections and Retin-A creams help restore skin turgor by either introducing collagen externally or stimulating blood flow and repair of the dermis, respectively.

The Hypodermis

The hypodermis (also called the subcutaneous layer or superficial fascia) is a layer directly below the dermis and serves to connect the skin to the underlying fascia (fibrous tissue) of the bones and muscles. It is not strictly a part of the skin, although the border between the hypodermis and dermis can be difficult to distinguish. The hypodermis consists of well-vascularized, loose, areolar connective tissue and adipose tissue, which functions as a mode of fat storage and provides insulation and cushioning for the integument.

Lipid Storage

The hypodermis is home to most of the fat that concerns people when they are trying to keep their weight under control. Adipose tissue present in the hypodermis consists of fat-storing cells called adipocytes. This stored fat can serve as an energy reserve, insulate the body to prevent heat loss, and act as a cushion to protect underlying structures from trauma. Where the fat is deposited and accumulates within the hypodermis depends on hormones (testosterone, estrogen, insulin, glucagon, leptin, and others), as well as genetic factors. Fat distribution changes as our bodies mature and age. Men tend to accumulate fat in different areas (neck, arms, lower back, and abdomen) than do women (breasts, hips, thighs, and buttocks). The body mass index (BMI) is often used as a measure of fat, although this measure is, in fact, derived from a mathematical formula that compares body weight (mass) to height. Therefore, its accuracy as a health indicator can be called into question in individuals who are extremely physically fit.

In many animals, there is a pattern of storing excess calories as fat to be used in times when food is not readily available. In much of the developed world, insufficient exercise coupled with the ready availability and consumption of high-calorie foods have resulted in unwanted accumulations of adipose tissue in many people. Although periodic accumulation of excess fat may have provided an evolutionary advantage to our ancestors, who experienced unpredictable bouts of famine, it is now becoming chronic and considered a major health threat. Recent studies indicate that a distressing percentage of our population is overweight and/or clinically obese. Not only is this a problem for the individuals affected, but it also has a severe impact on our healthcare system. Changes in lifestyle, specifically in diet and exercise, are the best ways to control body fat accumulation, especially when it reaches levels that increase the risk of heart disease and diabetes.

Pigmentation

The color of skin is influenced by a number of pigments, including melanin, carotene, and hemoglobin. Recall that melanin is produced by cells called melanocytes, which are found scattered throughout the stratum basale of the epidermis. The melanin is transferred into the keratinocytes via a cellular vesicle called a melanosome

Melanin occurs in two primary forms. Eumelanin exists as black and brown, whereas pheomelanin provides a red color. Dark-skinned individuals produce more melanin than those with pale skin. Exposure to the UV rays of the sun or a tanning salon causes melanin to be manufactured and built up in keratinocytes, as sun exposure stimulates keratinocytes to secrete chemicals that stimulate melanocytes. The accumulation of melanin in keratinocytes results in the darkening of the skin, or a tan. This increased melanin accumulation protects the DNA of epidermal cells from UV ray damage and the breakdown of folic acid, a nutrient necessary for our health and well-being. In contrast, too much melanin can interfere with the production of vitamin D, an important nutrient involved in calcium absorption. Thus, the amount of melanin present in our skin is dependent on a balance between available sunlight and folic acid destruction, and protection from UV radiation and vitamin D production.

It requires about 10 days after initial sun exposure for melanin synthesis to peak, which is why pale-skinned individuals tend to suffer sunburns of the epidermis initially. Dark-skinned individuals can also get sunburns, but are more protected than are pale-skinned individuals. Melanosomes are temporary structures that are eventually destroyed by fusion with lysosomes; this fact, along with melanin-filled keratinocytes in the stratum corneum sloughing off, makes tanning impermanent.

Too much sun exposure can eventually lead to wrinkling due to the destruction of the cellular structure of the skin, and in severe cases, can cause sufficient DNA damage to result in skin cancer. When there is an irregular accumulation of melanocytes in the skin, freckles appear. Moles are larger masses of melanocytes, and although most are benign, they should be monitored for changes that might indicate the presence of cancer

How To Treat All The Layer

The Layer system treats all of the seven layers of the skin. The system encourage applying a number of Natural active layers, one on top of the other; this method allows an accurate treatment and gives a perfect unblemished skin.

In each of the creams you should use there is a different active ingredient and every layer cares and treats in a different way. The layers system is based on separating between the active ingredients; this way you are provided with better results. Later on the book I will give examples with products you can buy everywhere that you can implement in your own layer system.

The secret of the layers system is the reaction between the active ingredients at the moment they contact the skin, this way each ingredient fills its part in the optimal way and various substances do not neutralize each other. True it would have been easier to get it all in one cream, but when you will test it, you will see that the amazing results were worth every minute of investment.

Chapter 2

The Layer System Foundation

Treating the inner layers of the skin is crucial to get real results from treating the skin. Using Mesotherapy as a tool to treat the deeper layer of the skin

What Is A Mesotherapy?

Meso means a middle And therapy - is a treatment. Which means that the method takes care of the middle of the skin, deep within the dermis. This method, which began to develop in 1952, is a penetrating therapeutic and Natural active ingredients into the subcutaneous skin thus effectively treats the skin. Use of natural materials is highly recommended and is an inseparable part in the treatment of mesotherapy, because the nutrients are absorbed into the skin and flow into the bloodstream.

This treatment has proven to give amazing results for:

- Scarring anywhere on the face or body

- Even out skin tone great for pigmentation

- Stimulate collagen production plump up skin – Drooping facial shape

- Anti aging, Wrinkles and fine lines

- Dull skin colour (due to less blood flow

- Skin feels dehydrated, and slightly rough

- Many more benefits to the skin

Because the skin-applied substances remain in the area for a long time, this method is excellent for treating almost all skin problems such as acne, seborrhea, scars, wrinkles and skin aging, as well as for the treatment of hair loss problems in the scalp.

Using a skin care roller is one of the most effective ways to treat with mesotherapy. The use of the roller has been known for more than 4000 years and has been developed in China as part of the acupuncture method that acts on the meridian points in the body and activates the energy of the chi, which is the energy of life in the treated area.

The use with a roller for the long-term causes the skin to be generally less sensitive to skin problems such as seborrhea, psoriasis, acne and sensitized or irritated skin.

What Are The Benefits Of Mesotherapy?

Roller with needles in different sizes according to the type of roller actually activates three mechanisms associated with anti-aging. The first: smoothing the needles on the skin actually causes a controlled skin injury. This process causes exfoliation that renews skin cells in all treated areas.

Meso Roller is making the efficiency of creams 30 to 100 times more....- It enable skin-care products to become easily absorbed into the skin. As a result, the products become more effective and the skin is better treated. The goal in any facial rejuvenation treatment is to make the fibroblasts in the skin produce more collagen. Collagen provides the scaffolding and support-read volume and lift here- for your skin. Slathering on cosmeceuticals will help to build some collagen-but only about 10 percent of a cream can be absorbed by the intact skin. Remember, your skin is the barrier between you and the outside environment, it cannot be too porous or you would evaporate! By creating micropunctures with a derma roller, about 80% of creams and serums will be absorbed. These tiny holes also stimulate the healing response in your skin.

The second important thing is that the roller opens microscopic holes in the skin At a depth of 0.3-2 mm (depending on the type of roller) and therefore all the treatment materials after the treatment penetrate to the depth of the skin and we get up to thirty times more activity from our cosmetics products The third thing is actually the wound itself, although this is a microscopic injury but the skin works in the repair process This process helps to rebuild the area treated with collagen and elastin, which are the basic building blocks of the skin, which flow from the body and contribute to the building and solidification of the treated area. Significant results can be achieved from multiple Treatment for wrinkles, scars and sores for all skin types, suitable for use at any age, easy to operate and gives cumulative results over time.

The Roller is the most effective tool known to science and cosmetic research. It is the cheapest treatment you can do to yourself in the comfort of your home with great results even compered to laser or IPL treatments. I suggest that you use the Roller at least once a week, on one regular day to maximize skin care efficiency. Derma Roller is the most powerful tool for mesotherapy and anti-aging. It was tested over the years for great results in preserving the skin and anti-aging

Using a roller decreases the sensitivity of the skin over time. It enforces its durability and lowering the inflammation in the treated areas

Derma Pen

Derma pen is one of the most popular and effective skin-care treatment alternatives to laser resurfacing, microdermabrasion, chemical peeling and other esthetic procedures. If you desire the look your skin would receive with laser treatments, microdermabrasion or chemical peels, but are not able or willing to endure the cost and/or the process, Microneedling may be the perfect option for you. This therapy is a minimally invasive skin rejuvenation treatment with quick recovery time and is designed to stimulate the body's natural collagen production. This is a unique way to address and correct:

- acne scars

- surgical scars

- chicken pox scars

- stretch marks

- wrinkles and upper lip lines

- hair loss

- hyperpigmentation

- lax skin

- sun damaged skin

- large pores and skin texture.

There is no risk of post-inflammatory hyper-pigmentation (pigmentation of the skin as a result of skin trauma) as the melanocytes and dermis remain intact during treatment. This is the major distinguishing safety feature when comparing microneedling and other invasive procedures that are used to treat deep lines and depressed scars, including laser resurfacing, deep chemical peels and dermabrasion all of which ablate the skin, making it thinner and progressively more prone to wrinkling.

Microneedling is a well established treatment option for acne scarring and pockmarks. It is a far more cost effective option than laser treatments and delivers very similar, if not better, results with repeated treatments. As the skin has a memory and will seek to return to its previous state, it is recommended to have 3-5 sessions every 3-4 weeks, and to repeat treatments over a period of one to two years. You will most likely experience a rosy complexion for a few hours following your treatment, looking like you've simply gotten a little too much sun. That will dissipate in the course of a few hours. By the next day, you'll be able to use product and make-up and no one will know that you've just had a facial rejuvenation treatment! You can even go back to work that very same day!

Your skin will become more firm, as it regains its elasticity, fine lines and wrinkles will be visibly reduced, pores become finer, circulation is stimulated and the overall condition of the skin improves for a more radiant complexion and youthful appearance.

How Does The Dermapen Work?

Dermapen excels when used as a treatment for fine lines and wrinkles. As the Dermapen glides over your skin, it creates micro-point punctures in the skin, the majority of which are simply pushing your pores open temporarily. This is perceived by the body as damage, which stimulates the release of growth factors that trigger the production of collagen and elastin. Your skin reacts to any injury by initiating the healing process. You encourage your skin to continue healing through this micro-needling process.

Your skin normally assumes that scars, stretch marks and wrinkles are repaired, but with the Dermapen micro-needling treatments, the skin is tricked into repairing itself. The process of skin remodeling can go on for months after each Dermapen treatment. Results can be seen within a week or even a few days.

The concept of micro-needling is based on the skin's ability to repair itself whenever it encounters physical damage such as cuts, burns and other abrasions. Immediately after an injury occurs our skin dissolves old damaged tissue and replaces it with new. DermaPen allows for controlled induction of the skin's self repair mechanism by creating micro "injuries" in the skin which triggers new collagen synthesis, yet does not pose the risk of permanent scarring. The result is smoother, firmer and younger looking skin. DermaPen's expertise is in optimising this process to improve results and minimise complications and discomfort.

How To Use A Roller Or Derma Pen

Using a roller with needles on your skin must sound terrifying, but believe me, it looks much worse than it really is. I have been derma rolling my skin for well over six months now with no adverse effects or harm to the skin. The biggest question I get is isn't it painful? For me? No. Remember though, everyone has a different pain tolerance and what it is completely fine for me may not be for you. If you're afraid of the pain, you can always use a numbing cream. In fact, most dermatologists or spas use numbing cream on clients before the procedure.

If you want to know how to derma roll on your own without hurting your skin, Here are the steps:

You will need:

- Skin cleanser

- Numbing cream

- Vitamin C serum

- Hyaluronic Acid

- Coconut oil (optional)

When To Derma Roll:

Do it at night because your skin will need time to repair itself. The wounds you create should heal within 15-30 minutes but derma rolling at night assures your skin gets the proper rest it needs. Avoid hot showers, exercise and makeup for at least 24 hours after since you don't want to irritate your already sensitive skin. But the number one tip of all is do not roll over active acne. Rolling over active areas of acne will only spread the bacteria to the rest of your face. Don't do it!

How Often To Derma Roll:

I usually derma roll once a week since it takes a bit of after care and you really want to allow your skin the chance to heal in between sessions. When I first started, I aimed for once every two weeks since I was just introducing my skin to this process, but as I progressed, I moved on to once a week. If you're concerned about not wearing make up the next day, try doing it on a weekend. I usually aim for Saturday.

How long should one treatment last? This is a very good question, but it varies for everyone. There should be no fixed time. However long it takes you to go over the affected area one time is how long it takes one treatment. Make sure to read and re-read the process of derma rolling in this ebook until you're confident enough to use the product.

What Kind Of Derma Roller To Get:

Derma roller needles can range in size from 0.25mm to 2.0mm. The size of the needle you choose is dependent on what skin issue you're trying to target. I use a 0.50mm needle since I'm not really trying to get rid of any major deep set wrinkles or acne scars;I'm just trying to improve my overall skin texture and target whatever fine lines may be starting to creep up. The 0.25mm to 0.75mm needle is great for targeting any acne scars or hyperpigmentation as well as any fine lines and wrinkles. I don't suggest using 1.0mm or higher at home since these deeply penetrate the skin, and if you use them incorrectly, you can damage the skin.

Sanitize Your Derma Roller:

Before you begin derma rolling, make sure to sanitize the roller properly. I do this by taking a 70% isopropyl alcohol and soaking my derma roller in the solution for at least 30 minutes.

Make sure you cover the head of the derma roller completely in alcohol.

Double Cleanse:

While this is soaking, I take the time to double cleanse my face. This step is super important as you want to make sure your skin is as clean as possible, so definitely take your time while cleansing to get rid of all of your makeup. If you want to take it a step further, you can also go for a triple cleanse and use a cleansing water to make sure you've gotten rid of all leftover over makeup or residue. After your face is all nice and clean, remove your derma roller from the solution and set it aside to dry. At this point, I take an alcohol soaked cotton pad and gently swipe it across my face. Before you freak out about using alcohol on your face, let me explain why I do this: Since you're putting tiny needles on our face, it's essential that you have your skin as clean as possible. Using the alcohol takes it a step further and rids the skin of any possible germs or bacteria.

Hydrate With A Derma Roll Serum:

Post-cleansing with the alcohol pad, I use a super hydrating serum on my face. I usually go for a pure hyaluronic acid as this will help to hydrate and soothe the skin as I derma roll over it. I tend to go a bit heavy handed with the application because I want the serum to take its time to absorb while I'm derma rolling. The serum also helps to create a slippery surface for the derma roller so it can glide over the skin much easier.

If your serum absorbs before you're done derma rolling, no worries! Just add a bit more so you can complete your session. You're going to look super shiny during this process but it's worth it.

How To Derma Roll

Derma Roll Section

Here's the fun part! Derma roll section by section. You can start anywhere you like but you'll want to go over the cheeks, the forehead, the nose, the chin, the lips (this will create a temporary plumping of the lips) and the jaw line. If you're brave, you can also derma roll by the corner of your eyes (where crows feet would usually occur) but you want to be super gentle in this area.

Derma Roll Eye

Roll it in several different directions on each section of your face: from left to right, top to bottom, and then diagonal both ways. Roll it in each direction at least 4 to 8 times. This ensures that you're targeting every part of the skin.

If you want, after you're done with the first session, you can apply more serum and go back over it a second time to get any areas you may have missed. The most important tip during this process: Lift the derma roller as you change directions! Dragging the roller in a new direction will only work to harm the skin. Also, apply a gentle amount of pressure and don't overdo it.

In total, derma rolling takes about 5-10 minutes (spend at least a minute on each section of the face) so it's a super short process.

Immediately After Derma Rolling:

Right after derma rolling you're going to be red as a lobster but don't panic — it's temporary. Any redness that you may experience should go away within 30 minutes to an hour. But it really depends on how sensitive your skin is and how aggressive you go with the derma roller, so you may be a bit red the next day, but this will also go away.

Your skin will also feel tight and like it has a slight sunburn, but this is completely normal. Don't forget to sanitize your derma roller and allow it to dry after use. You want to do this before and after every single session to make sure you're keeping it as clean as possible.

The next day:

My skin always feels so smooth the day after derma rolling and it ends up having a much more even and glowy look to it. But remember: The long term results are not instantaneous (nothing in skin care really is), and if you're targeting more deep set acne scars or wrinkles, you'll want to be consistent with derma rolling. If you are, you should see results after a couple of sessions. Beauty takes time!

Chapter 3

Importance Of Natural Products

Chemical Products Awareness

It is very important to use natural products because the ingredients goes right to the skin and mixing with the blood stream. With so many skincare products on the market today, how can you determine which ones are the best for your skin? You can easily narrow down your choices by making an effort to use only all-natural products. By understanding the importance of natural skincare, you will be able to see just how beneficial natural products are when compared to their chemical-laden counterparts.

According to The National Institute of Occupational Safety & Health, there are over 800 toxic ingredients being added to skincare products every day. 300 of those were proven to cause developmental abnormalities, while over 700 were shown to produce acute toxic effects. Many of these toxins contain particulates that are so small; they can be absorbed by the brain and body 3 times more quickly than water.

Skincare products that contain all-natural ingredients are designed to complement your skin's sophisticated system. The skin has a remarkable ability to heal and maintain itself, but only when it is given the proper nutrients. Because the skin is the largest bodily organ, it can absorb any and everything you apply to it directly into the bloodstream. Even though you may follow a healthy diet, applying skincare products that contain known toxins can affect your health in detrimental ways, causing you to become ill.

There are numerous studies that have proven the link between illness and synthetic chemicals. Using skincare products that contain synthetics can result in headaches, disrupted hormone levels, breathing disorders, and even cancer. With so many dangers associated with synthetics, why would anyone want to use products that contain them?

There is a simple answer: because they provide instant gratification. Many chemical-based skincare products can instantly reduce the appearance of wrinkles and even fade sunspots, but they do so through dangerous means. These products starve the skin of oxygen, and increase photo-sensitivity (makes the skin sensitive to the sunlight). Year's later, extensive use of these products can increase the risk of sunspots and cause premature aging: the very things the products were designed to prevent.

Even though chemical-based products have been tested and proven to be 'safe', they can still cause harm. A product can be labeled as 'non-toxic' if 50% or less of lab animals it was tested on died within 2 weeks. Children's shampoos that are labeled as a 'no tears' formula contain anesthetics to numb the burning sensation the eyes would experience with normal shampoo.

When using Mesotherapy it is ALSO important to use Natural and effective products and not to include harmful chemicals that reaches into the blood stream.

Many body lotions also contain dangerous chemicals, such as artificial fragrances and colors. They may also contain ingredients such as mineral oils and parabens that can clog the skin's pores and cause breakouts. Natural skincare products allow the skin to breathe, which will help prevent acne, rashes, and other irritations.

To ensure your skin receives proper nourishment without harmful chemicals, only use products that contain plant-derived ingredients and are free of synthetic fertilizers and pesticides. Products that state they contain the extracts of organically-grown ingredients are the best choice for proper skincare. By paying close attention to the products you apply to your skin, you can keep it at its healthiest and allow it to look younger for longer.

Chapter 4

Pharma Vs Professional Products

Get The Real Stuff

I'm often asked, "What is the difference between Pharma (over the counter) products sold at drugstores or department stores compared to professional products like yours?" "Do professional products work better?"

The simplest answer is yes. BUT, the truth is that there really is a difference between Pharma (over the counter) products and professional products that you purchase from an Aestheticians. The biggest difference is in the active ingredients. These ingredients are the main reason you should be purchasing the product. Actually not so much the ingredients but what results these ingredients will give you.

Pharma (over the counter) products are sold at drugstores and do not contain high dosage of active ingredients. Professional products are sold at Aestheticians only and contain high percentage of active ingredients like Retinol and AHA BHA Amino acids and glycolic lactic etc acids

The old adage says it best: you get what you pay for. When it comes to skin care products, professionals agree that this holds true. The sea of over-the-counter products at the drugstore is overwhelming to shoppers. Just like the foods you eat for the nourishment of your body, it is important to know the ingredients and origin of the topical products used on your skin.

Why Are Active Ingredients Important?

These are the ingredients that MAKE a change in the skin. Some of the conditions or concerns that most consumers are trying to correct: Hyperpigmentation, Melasma, Fine lines & Wrinkles, Hydration, Sun Spots ext.

Certain ingredients don't even begin to have an effect in the skin unless they are at a certain percentage or concentration. Other ingredients don't do anything for the skin unless they are used in a delivery system that can actually penetrate the stratum corneum (the upper layers of your skin). And certain ingredients like Vitamin C come in many different forms but only some forms are recognized by the skin, and THEN they need to be used at the proper pH or stabilized so they don't oxidize and actually make your skin worse.

There are several reasons that Pharma products can never give you the true results you desire. First, Pharma products are sold in huge retail chains so the manufacturers are selling to millions of customers. These retailers assume that clients know what type of skin they have and what types of products they should be using. They are able to keep the costs down because 1) they are using a very low percentage of the active ingredients and 2) Most of the inactive ingredients are things you can't even pronounce and probably don't really want to put on your face.

These large manufacturers mean well, but they don't want to put enough of an active ingredient in a product to cause too much of a difference in the skin. Why? Because if they put too much then someone can have a really bad reaction and they can get sued. Ingredients like glycolic acid and retinol and benzoyl peroxide MUST be prescribed by an esthetician so that you know how often to use them, what time of day, and when not to use. For example, retinol and acids should ONLY be used at night and if you're not using something with SPF every day, there's a real chance you can burn. Professional strength retinol products should generally be started every other night so the skin can build up a tolerance and then usage can be increased to every night. There is no one in Rite-Aid to analyze your skin, tell you how to get the results you want and how to use the products. This is how they keep costs down.

Here are the reasons why professional products are more effective and will deliver better results than drugstore or department store products.

Pharma products ONLY work with the outer most layer of the skin. This is the skin you see when looking in the mirror. So when you use Pharma products you are applying the product and it just sits on the surface of the skin. It will not penetrate any deeper! Bummer RIGHT! I know. Think of all the money spent over the years on products that just work on the surface. Pharma products have so many fillers, parabens, dyes, fragrance ext and they are most likely watered down. Look at your products, what is the first ingredient? This is what your product mostly consists of.

Now when you use Professional products they actually penetrate through the Epidermis all the way to Dermis where your collagen, elastin, and new skin cells reside... This is what we want to target with skin care products!!! We want to get rid of any unhealthy skin cells that cause pigmentation problems or uneven skin texture. You want to BOOST collagen, elastin and speed up cell turnover, this is what makes healthy skin.

When our collagen and elastin are broken down we will not have that tight plump looking skin. It is very hard to replace collagen and elastin after it's been damaged, this is why you should be using a cosmeceutical on a daily basis so you can preserve and protect what you have!

One the BIGGEST reasons consumers purchase Pharma products are because they think they cannot afford medical grade Professional products. This is not true. Most Pharma products you get from the drug store, department stores, independent cosmetic sales consultants or even a mall kiosk are often the same price or more expensive. You end up using more of the product and replacing it sooner. Which means more $$$$! Also Professional products are more affordable because they have a higher concentration of great quality ingredients, they last longer because you do not use as much, and they don't pay for T.V. commercials or big advertising campaigns.

Are Professional Products Worth The Money?

Pharma skin care products are often made with lower quality, less expensive ingredients. Therefore, when comparing Pharma products to professional products, it may seem like Pharma products is less expensive. However, be mindful of how frequently you're purchasing Pharma products, and you may discover it is not the cheaper option. Professional products have more concentrated active ingredients than Pharma products, so a little bit goes a long way, meaning fewer trips to the store. With the added benefit of positive results, the professional products make the most sense for your pocketbook.

Professional products are very concentrated so a little goes a long way. Ultimately they end up being a better value for your money as they last longer than Pharma products, but most important, they give you the results you want.

Important Information To Know:

Two products can have the exact same list of ingredients, and one will be highly effective while the other could be completely useless. The difference is the concentration of those ingredients. One product may use a very small amount while the other uses a clinically active level. Unfortunately for you, the consumer, there is no way to understand the difference. This is because all ingredients are supposed to be listed in order of the concentration used, but for ingredients with a concentration less than 1% they can be listed in any order. There's a big difference between an ingredients used at .01% versus 1%, but you would never know it from the label on the bottle, tube or jar.

Since skin care formulas are proprietary, cheap products can easily disguise themselves as looking like quality products–especially if fancy packaging is used. You must choose a skin care company that you trust. The credentials of the company as well as positive results experienced by real customers make all of the difference in skin care.

If you truly want to improve the appearance in your skin, I think there is no better place to purchase your skin care products than through a reputable skin care professional.

Chapter 5

Seven Steps To Ageless Beauty

The layer system is built on seven steps of treatment for day and for the night, you can do just part of the steps but you will get less results with the system.

How To Treat The Face With The Layer System

Step 1:

The First Step is Cleansing with natural products. Cleansers remove all traces of makeup and pollution. All skin care treatment start with an exfoliate Product that is recommended at least once a day. Balancing exfoliates speed up the epidermis' natural renewal process and the reconstruction of the epidermal shield, they are easy to rinse and remove impurities, dead skin cells and regulates excessive sebum secretion.

The active ingredients initiate the beauty treatment and leave the skin soft and refreshed. These products are used in the first stage of every skin care regime and are used every day in the morning and in the evening.

Products to use: AHA BHA and glycolic and lactic acid cleansers

Exfoliating As The Key
For Skin Renewal Process

Exfoliation makes your skin glow and may even help to prevent wrinkles. Many of us know the benefits of exfoliation in whisking away complexion-dulling dead skin cells. But it does more than that, says Holly Sherrard, education manager for Dermalogica Canada. 'Exfoliating increases cell turnover to reveal newer, healthier skin cells, plus it decreases blackheads, minimises hyperpigmentation and fine lines, and imparts an all-over healthy glow.' It also helps with hydration. 'Cells transitioning from below the skin's surface to the topmost layer bring with them essential lipids and moisture,' she says.

'Exfoliating increases cell turnover to reveal newer, healthier skin cells, plus it decreases blackheads, minimises hyperpigmentation and fine lines, and imparts an all-over healthy glow.'

As we age, our natural cell turnover rate decreases. Adding additional skincare support into our routine can help us maintain that youthful glow longer. One of these is exfoliation. Exfoliation involves the removal of the oldest layer of dead skin cells on the skin's outermost surface, and it should be your go-to skin care step to revive dull looking skin, and regain a youthful, glowing complexion.

What Is Exfoliation?

Natural homemade clay facial masks at home. Before you even think about exfoliating, you need to know what it is and what it does. This is the process of removing the dead skin cells from the body, so your newer, fresher skin cells are left at the top. Your skin feels smoother and looks much more radiant that it did just before.

You'll also find that it can clear the pores of all the dirt and oils much easier, so you're left with cleaner skin ready for your day or night ahead.

Exfoliation can also rejuvenate the skin. During the winter, it is easy to want to hide away. Your skin may not get as much sun as it needs, and it starts to look dull. By creating a beauty routine that you follow throughout the year, you will have sun-ready skin all the time.

Most people will exfoliate their faces on a daily basis. Many facial cleansing products come with microbeads that help to clear away the dead skin cells. However, most will forget about the rest of their body. It can leave dull looking shoulders and legs when it comes to bikini weather or those gorgeous evening gowns.

Exfoliating can also help make dry skin look smoother and softer. You get rid of the flakes that appear. However, you may need to work your exfoliating routine in with your moisturising routine to really get the best benefit.

Why Your Skin Needs More Exfoliation

Exfoliation is important. It's the key to healthy skin. Your skin does this naturally every day as a part of its normal renewal process. Helping your skin exfoliate with a daily skin cleansing process further aids it to remove any lingering dead skin cells to help your skin be at its best.

But how often is enough? Well, it depends. The overall benefits show the more exfoliation, generally the better (but don't overdo it!). Many try to eek out it a few times a week for those with normal or combination skin and less frequently for people with sensitive skin.

Many dermatologists recommend daily exfoliation (twice every day!) as be a key part of your regular daily skin care routine. Daily gentle exfoliation should be an essential part of your skin's regular cleansing process. Like we said, the more regular exfoliation generally the better. However, for those with sensitive skin types or those who haven't exfoliated properly for some time might only be able to handle exfoliation once or twice a week initially, but gentle exfoliation can be gradually increased to a daily frequency. How your skin responds also depends on your skin's condition.

If your skin is oily or you exercise often, daily gentle exfoliation will also help remove any oils that could be trapped with any lingering dead skin cells. If you have mature, flaking, or dull skin, (often times caused by a buildup of dead skin layers caused by lowered hormones from menopause), or have been under stress, adding an exfoliation boost a few times per week to the daily exfoliation routine with a chemical exfoliant such as glycolic acid may be necessary and quite helpful. As with anything related to you body, the best way to is to introduce daily exfoliation or to add the exfoliation boost is to do so gently and gradually to work with your skin's natural functions.

Here's the Ten reasons why you should exfoliate your skin:

1. Exfoliation Makes Skin Smoother

Dead cells love piling up on the surface of your skin, making it rougher to the touch. Then, there are wrinkles. They make your skin fold and crease. A little bit of exfoliation will smooth everything out. Yep, even wrinkles. It won't remove them completely, but it'll make them look smaller. Exfoliating removes the rough, dry dead skin cells sitting on top of your skin. Once those are gone, skin has a much smoother feel and appearance.

2. And Brighter

You know what else all those dead cells do to your skin? They rob it of its natural glow. If your skin's been dull and lackluster lately, now you know what to blame. Exfoliation helps remove dirt, debris, excess oil and dulling skin cells that make your skin appear old and wrinkled. So, exfoliate away!

3. Evens Out Skin Tone

Exfoliating the darker body patches daily with a gentle body scrub can help you get smooth and even-toned skin in no time. Exfoliation is not merely a cosmetic requirement—it's a hygiene must. Exfoliation gets rid of accumulated dead cells, opens clogged pores, and promotes tighter and lighter skin. It's easy to see how exfoliating can help even out your skin tone. Many inconsistencies in your skin may be the result of dead skin cells that haven't been shed yet and exfoliation helps speed up that process. Making sure your outer layer of skin cells is healthy and new will help you look and feel better.

4. Rids Our Skin Of Pimples, Blackheads & Whiteheads

Acne-prone skin sheds skin cells more rapidly than normal or dry skin. However, those skin cells can get stuck on the skin surface, irritating pores. Exfoliating cleans away dead skin cells that clog pores and hair follicles. If your skin's producing way too much oil than it needs, some of it will remain trapped in your pores. Together with dead skin cells, they clog the pores. That's a recipe for pimples, blackheads, whiteheads… all forms of acne, basically. Guess how you get rid of them? By exfoliating those pores, of course! Getting rid of blackheads, breakouts and all is great. But, wouldn't it be even better if you didn't have to deal with them in the first place? Exfoliate those pores regularly and you won't have to. The gunk won't have the time to accumulate in there fast enough.

5. Slows Down The Aging Process

Did you know that your skin renews itself every month or so? When it's young. As it gets older, it needs a little helping hand to make that happen. Enter exfoliation. It speeds up the process, helping your skin get rid of old and damaged cells and replacing them with newer and healthier ones more quickly.

The skin's natural exfoliation process helps to keep skin looking young and wrinkle-free. However, as we age, that process slows down. As you incorporate exfoliation into your skincare routine, you are tricking the skin into acting younger again, speeding up skin renewal.

6. Reduce Appearance Of Dark Spots & Age Spots

Those skin cells on the surface are the oldest. The most sun damaged. That's why they create darker spots on your face. Then, there are freckles, melasma, and well… there can be 100 reasons why your skin tone is darker in certain places and lighter in others. Whatever the cause, getting rid of those top dead cells will lighten those dark spots. Exfoliating aids in speeding up cell turnover, they key to fading brown spots and discolouration. The more you remove the damaged cells on the skin's surface, the faster the new, healthy cells will move up to replace them.

7. Shrinks Pores (Kind Of)

Ok, the size of your pores is genetically determined, so you can't shrink it. But, when your pores are clogged, the crap in there will stretch them out, making them look a lot larger than they naturally are. So, if your pores are the size of an orange, you know what to do. Exfoliate!

8. Relieves Dry/Itchy Skin

Dry skin means you have a buildup of dry skin cells. Even though layering on a heavy moisturiser may feel like you are rehydrating skin, that moisturiser cannot get through the layer of dry skin cells to actually moisturise the skin underneath. Exfoliating will remove that layer, allowing your moisturiser to heal and hydrate your skin.

9. Increases Natural Collagen Production

By exfoliating, removing the top layer of dead skin cells, skin is tricked into producing new cells which helps stimulate new collagen production. This helps to improve smoothness and reduce the appearance of wrinkles/fine lines!!

10. Allows Moisturisers To Do Their Job

By removing the dead skin cells that can be clogging your pores and blocking your skin from absorbing that oh-so-important treatment product, exfoliating can help you get the most out of your anti-aging products. You can use the best skincare products in the world, but if they meet a thick wall of dead skin cells, they won't be able to penetrate deep enough to do their job. So, if you want to see results quickly (or at all), remove all obstacles from their way.

Step 2:

The second Step takes care of the deep layers of the skin with The Mesotherapy Serums that are pure and Powerful Cellular Regenerators. Their main active ingredients are Hyaluronic Acid and other amino acids or short peptides and advanced active ingredients. They are designed to treat specific skin imbalances like pigmentation, firmness and moistness. The bio-mimetic serums can be used alone, or mixed together used preferably before the Active layers.

Derma Roller Machine can be used to optimize their effect on the skin. Look for products that are based on cutting-edge bio/nano technology and work perfectly with all other products. Good serums activates cellular regeneration process, protects against the harmful effects of free radicals and boosts the skin's protective functions while improving epidermal moisture and tone. The series is enriched with botanical extracts, and additional active natural ingredients to repair flaws and nourish the skin.

Products to use: Hyaluronic acid and peptides

Hyaluronic Acid

Hyaluronic Acid is a product that cushions the skin and gives it its smoothness.

Hyaluronic Acid (Hyaluronic Acid, Sodium Hyaluronate, HA) has many benefits and is one of the most interesting ingredients in skin care, specifically. Naturally found in the body, hyaluronic acid secures moisture and creates fullness youthful skin naturally abounds with hyaluronic acid.

The more hyaluronic acid you can get into your skin, the younger and fresher you'll look—and now there are newer, and better, ways to load up. Hyaluronic acid is a little complicated. First, it's not actually an acid. It's a sugar. Also, it's a sponge. Every molecule can hold 1,000 times its weight in water. But one thing about hyaluronic acid has always been 100 percent straightforward: It's a skin-care star. In serums and creams, it smooths and plumps (temporarily); as an injectable, it erases wrinkles (for months). Let's be honest, though: We've taken hyaluronic acid for granted for a while. Sure, it's great stuff, always welcome at the party. But when's the last time you were like, "Guys, hyaluronic acid is here!" That's about to change. A fresh crop of innovations has us taking a new look at the old standby. Chemists and dermatologists are using hyaluronic acid in unprecedented ways to make skin dewier, firmer, and a whole lot awesomer.

Why Hyaluronic Acid Is Important For The Skin?

As we age, skin moisture can drop significantly, which makes the skin lose elasticity and expose the signs of aging on the skin. Hyaluronic acid plays a critical role in skin health with its unique ability to hold in moisture (1000 ml of water per gram of hyaluronic acid).

1. Hyaluronic acid is also a "smart nutrient" as it can adjust its moisture absorption rate based on the humidity — relative to the season and the climate.

2. Benefits of Hyaluronic Acid and UVB Sun Protection- One of the most skin damaging elements are UVB rays from the sun. Hyaluronic acid benefits the skin as it protects the skin from UVB rays (and the scavenging reactive oxygen species they generate), which can cause sunspots.

3. Hyaluronic Acid Research- Researchers have found Hyaluronic Acid supplementation to be directly correlated to measured increases in skin moisture.

Microscopic skin surface analysis shows increased skin smoothness, and amelioration of wrinkles.

Difference Between Home Use Hyaluronic Acid To Those You Inject By Doctors

Hyaluronic acid can be injected into the dermis of the skin to fill and plump, a technique more commonly known as dermal fillers. Hyaluronic acid can also be applied topically and is a key ingredient in many serums and creams. While the molecule is too large to get down into the dermis layer, there are benefits to using it on the skin's surface. It acts as a moisturiser through its water-attracting properties. This means it draws water into the skin to keep it hydrated, supple and functioning effectively as a barrier.

This will produce a temporary improvement in lines and wrinkles. However, the hyaluronic acid will not penetrate beneath the skin and add volume in the way that dermal fillers do. Serums will make your skin look brighter and smoother but will not fill in lines or folds. Dermal fillers are precisely placed with a cannula or needle and last 1-2 years in the tissue. With regard to your hands, Voluma and Radiesse both work very well for covering up skeletal or very thin hands.

Peptides And Its Benefits

Peptides is small molecules that penetrate the skin and helps him rebuild himself. Peptides, a fancy name for short chain amino acids, are one of the newest innovations in professional skincare. You might be familiar with amino acids as "the building blocks of protein", body builders and athletes have been ingesting them for years to enhance their physiques and build muscle. In fact, our bodies are made up of thousands of amino acids that help our cells to function in everything that we do. So, what's that got to do with your skin?

Our bodies naturally produce about 20 different amino acids. Those amino acids link together to form short chains called peptides. When a peptide chain consists of over 50 amino acids, it forms a protein such as collagen. However, that's not exactly how peptides work on your skin. Studies have shown that peptides actually change the membrane structure of skin cells, making it easier to absorb the ingredients in your skincare serums and lotions. In addition, peptides send a message to cells below the top layers of skin, telling them to produce more collagen. The result is that skin can recapture and maintain its youthful appearance in a way that is similar to the results of Botox.

Peptides, work best when applied topically within a cream or serum that contains other active ingredients. This is because most peptide molecules are too large to penetrate the skin on their own but, research shows that when combined with other active ingredients, the molecule is much more effective. That being said, it's important to only use peptide containing products that are stable and have an appropriate delivery system.

Are Peptides Stable?

One of the reasons that peptides work so effectively is because of their ability to easily bond with other molecules, preferably those in your skin. If a peptide is poorly stabilized they will end up bonding with the inactive ingredients in your lotion or serum instead, making them useless. This is one reason why high quality products, such as PCA Skin Exlinea Peptide Smoothing Skin Serum, are worth splurging on.

Consistency is Key

Another factor to keep in mind is the delivery system. Most peptide molecules are too large to penetrate the skin. Instead, they rely on changing the chemical composition of the skin membrane in order to send signals to skin cells below the epidermis. It's important that the cream, lotion or serum that is being used allows maximum penetration of product and is not too thick. A high quality product will come in a cream or serum that is lightweight and absorbs rapidly into the skin. With a high efficacy rate and the ability to produce significant results without invasive measures, there's no denying the power of peptides.

Step 3 :

The third step is one of the most important steps in the treatment and takes care of the skin layer which produces the Melanin and skin pigmentation. These creams contain high concentrations of active ingredients, amino acids such as retinol, alpha and beta hydroxide and other whitening agents, to balance and purify the epidermis and preserve all the benefits of previous treatments. They contain amino acids to replenish the skins proteo-lipidic film after exfoliation and prepare the skin for the products that are applied during the next Stage.

The special formula acts to suppress the melanin production, whiten pigmentation, stimulate gentle peel and accelerates the natural renewal of skin cells. The procedure not only helps prevent the formation of wrinkles but guards against signs of premature aging, treats the upper layers of the skin as well as the deeper ones and even enhances the other products. When you start enjoying the Luminescence series you will notice immediate improvement in how your skin looks and feels with improved hydration, increased firmness and elasticity, and a smoother, more refined appearance.

Products to use: Retinol AHA, BHA, glycolic acid lactic etc

What Is Retinol And What Can It Do For My Skin?

Have you been thinking about introducing retinol into your beauty regimen?

Vitamin A (retinol) is a term used for a group of compounds which can be broken down into more potent compounds, called retinoids. Although the terms vitamin A, retinol, and retinoid often are used interchangeably, each has its own distinctive actions and regulations. For example, some forms of retinol can be used freely in cosmetics, while others (retinoids) can be obtained only by prescription.

What do we need vitamin A for?

Vitamin A plays a key role in the development and integrity of the skin, and also the eye and nerve cells, and immune functions. We get dietary vitamin A from oily fish, eggs, butter, cheese and some fruit and vegetables, like carrots. Deficiency in oral vitamin A can result in damage to the skin and eyes, but in the developed world, vitamin A deficiency is extremely rare. While we need adequate dietary vitamin A intake, this doesn't seem to protect the skin against ageing changes or sun damage, and for this we need to look at topical or cream versions of vitamin A to see beneficial results.

What are the benefits of retinol?

Retinol works to:

- stimulate collagen

- improve skin texture

- reduce fine lines and wrinkles

- strengthen ageing skin

- reduce sun damage

- reduce pigmentation and age spots

- reduce pore size

- reduce skin laxity

- reduce skin roughness

When should I not use Retinol?

Retinol products are not suitable for use if you are pregnant, planning a pregnancy in the next three months, or breast-feeding (due to the vitamin A content). I recommend taking a break from retinol products three days before any facial peels or Dermapen (micro-needling procedure), and for one week after peels or Dermapen procedures. Stop retinol products for a few days before and after facial waxing to avoid irritation.

AHA/Alpha Hydroxy Acids

AHA stands for Alpha Hydroxy Acid. These acids are a category of chemical combinations which contains with carboxylic acid alternated with hydroxyl group of the adjoining carbon. Alpha Hydroxy Acids are very popular for skin care treatment and are using widely in the entire cosmetics application. These forms of acids are sometimes found in different products that are used to minimize wrinkles, aging purposes and to get better look of the face. The acids are well known and are using in the cosmetic industry to get and to reduce various skin problems, and to get a comprehensive look and freshness of skin. These acids perforate your skin very clearly and easily due to that it has been gaining popularity day by day. There are several benefits of AHAs for the purpose of your skin. Let's have a brief look on it.

1. Remove dead skin cells

Alpha Hydroxy Acids is very good which works as a chemical remover for your skin, which helps you to loose and to get rid of dark cells from the top layer of your skin. The acids are really awesome and very much effective than any other coarse chemical removers, for instance cloths and or sponge.

2. Prevent your skin form Sun Damage

Your skin can be damaged by san light, your skin can look blemish and other problems can be seen and the outcomes are hyper-pigmentation and patch on skin. Though, a flesh-toned cosmetic stick can disguise the patch mark on your skin but it does not precise to make clear the quality of your skin.

3. Grows Assimilation

The exterior waste, dull and dead skin cells hamper the ability of your skin in absorbing the vigorous components for your skin protection serums and creams. In this condition AHAs detach these layer stakes to uncover the primary cells. It is also helpful in optimizing your skin level immersion so that you can get the extremely good outcome from your skin care cream.

4. AHAs Reduces Wrinkles

In accordance with University of Maryland Medical Center, AHAs are very much helpful to reduce the acuteness of the layers of skin and wrinkles in a short period of time. You can find out AHAs in different products of body and face creams, such as sunscreen, anti-aging creams, acne creams, and several related shampoos.

5. Escape from Damaged Skin

Alpha Hydroxy Acid for Skin helps to decamp to top damaged skin surface and help to regain the vigorous skin cells. AHAs also help to increase the production of collagen in your body and intensify the protein which push and make a solid resistance for the surface of your skin.

6. Rise blood flow to the skin

In accordance with Harvard Medical School, using AHAs increase the blood flow to your skin and helps you to reduce wrinkles and crumples, the results you get a natural and bright toned skin and block in increasing the dead cells which is the cause of your dull skin.

7. Get an Overall Fresh Look

One of the most important benefits of AHAs is very embryonic in reducing dark spots on your skin, minimize blackheads and very good for acne. Alpha Hydroxy Acid for Skin are commonly safe and secure for various people, who have sensitive skin. It helps fine refinement of your skin and gives an overall fresh look.

8. Overall Protection of your skin

If you use it on a regular basis it helps you to exfoliate your outermost surface of the skin and makes your skin smoother, glowing, reduce acne, wrinkle and dark skin or tan. You can use it to get the fastest outcome. People who desire to get smooth and tanned skin can use AHAs, using AHAs based creams work very nicely for protecting the overall look of your skin.

9. Works As Anti-Aging Agent

Creams consist with alpha hydroxy acids are the best routes to get rid of skin aging. Regular using can give you a very good result in a month or less time the amount of improvement you want. Whether you're looking for good skin care products, such as creams or lotions, then you can buy the products which contain AHAs acids and make sure to purchase an extra sunscreen. Yes, sometimes you think that AHAs can unmask new skin to sun damage but a right sun screen is truly in need to protect aging for your skin.

BHA/Beta Hydroxy Acids

BHA, also known as salicylic acid, is beta hydroxy acid - a derivative of aspirin. Beta hydroxy acid has several uses - it's the key active in Pepto-Bismol - but in skincare it is mainly used to fight acne, thanks to its anti-inflammatory, anti-microbial and exfoliating properties. Since it has the ability to penetrate the skin it offers deep pore exfoliation as well as acting on the skin's surface. Percentages of 0.5 to 2 per cent are usually gentle enough for at-home use.

Benefits of Beta Hydroxy Acid

1. Keep oily shine at bay

Beta Hydroxy acid, naturally dissolves oils in the skin. The fact that this acid is oil soluble, means it penetrates deep into the dermis, breaking down keratin (protein) and sebum (oil), that builds up overtime in the skin's pores, It mops up excess oil, making it the perfect treatment for an oily face.

2. Balances a Combination Skin

If you are plagued with pimples, or suffer from an oily T zone or comedones, then chances are you have a combination skin.

Beta Hydroxy Acid is the perfect prep treatment for this particular skin type, it liquefies sebum and softens the skins tissues, so that it is ready for comedone extraction.

3. Perfect Acne Treatment

Not only are Beta Hydroxy acids extremely deep cleansing, but they also help to break the cycle of infection. They stop acne bacteria in it's tracks, neutralizing P-Acnes bacteria in the pores, making it the perfect treatment for acneic skin conditions.

4. A dehydrated skins best friend

If your skin ever feel like it is one size to small, then chances are it's dehydrated. Applying a low concentration of Beta Hydroxy acid, will significantly help to boost moisture retention in the skins tissues.

5. Exfoliating Treatment

Did you know that as we age, our cellular turnover starts to slow down? Stubborn skin cells stick together, often making the skin dry and flaky. Beta hydroxy acid is the perfect exfoliating treatment, helping to encourage stubborn epidermal cells to shed.

So just to recap and look at the benefits of this awesome ingredient:

- It is the perfect treatment for a dry, thirsty skin

- It shows a significant decrease, in the appearance of fine lines and wrinkles

- A possible anti wrinkle cure, it can help to visibly improve skin tone and texture

- It can help to reduce signs of photoaging, reducing the appearance of liver spots and irregular pigmentation, caused by damaging UV rays

- When used correctly, Beta Hydroxy acids can work as an anti-inflammatory, helping to treat rosacea and other sensitive skin conditions

So I think you'd agree, this is one serious skin care ingredient, you may want to consider including in your skin care routine.

Step 4:

This products are the Forth Step of the treatment and strengthening the eyes and lips area. The eye area is the most sensitive areas in the human body; sometime it may present specific or temporary imbalances that require targeted treatment and both immediate and lasting results.

These products are from the new generation of creams with formula that its active principles will attack the causes and eliminate the problem whether its puffiness, wrinkles or dryness. Use twice a day for nice relaxed and smooth eye area.

Products to use: Shea butter, natural soothing creams & argilanine peptide

Shea Butter And Its Benefits

Shea butter comes from the African shea tree. The fat of the nut is processed to make butter, which is heralded around the world for its many different benefits to users. While widely known as one of nature's richest moisturizers, some of shea butter's lesser-known benefits include the fact that it contains antioxidants, is anti-inflammatory, and has healing qualities.

What makes Shea butter an extraordinary skin care and an amazing body healer is its richness in precious constituents, which include unsaturated fats with a large proportion of "unsaponifiables" components, essential fatty acids, phytosterols, vitamin E and D, provitamin A and allantoin.

All these are natural and make Shea butter a superfood for your skin (and hair), but that is not all it can do for you because it is:

- Antioxidant

- Anti-inflammatory

- Deeply moisturizing

- Skin strengthening

- Skin protecting

- UV protecting

- Skin regenerating

- Minor cuts and burns healing

- Muscle ache healing

- Physical endurance enhancer

- Wrinkles, fine lines and scars repairing

- Stimulating for the superficial microcirculation

- Collagen production stimulating (makes the skin stronger, more supple and younger)

Due to all of these benefits, shea butter is used in beauty and health regimes around the world. Not only does it moisturize skin, but it can also reduce the appearance of scars, fine lines, and stretch marks. Many make-up manufacturers use it in their cosmetics. It also works as a natural soother for skin irritations such as sunburns, eczema, psoriasis, and, in some cases, rosacea. However, shea butter's use is not just limited to the world of health and beauty. Since shea butter can soften and condition leather and wood, many musicians use it on animal skin drums and leather tuning straps. In Africa, it is also used in cooking. To get the best benefits out of your shea butter, make sure that you are using unrefined or grade A butter. Lower grades will have lower results.

Argilanine Peptide And Its Benefits

Peptides are found in many effective anti-aging skin care products. While there is no singular, miracle ingredient that will give you those instant, youthful results we all wish for, peptides are an extremely important ingredient to look for in your wrinkle fighting creams, serums, and under eye products.

What are Peptides?

Peptides are formed by chains of amino acids that are the building blocks of skin proteins. When peptides are created by a long chain of amino acids, they become proteins. Forming peptides from a short chain of amino acids allows them to penetrate the outer layer of our skin and send signals to our cells to remind them how to function properly.

The most infamous protein naturally found in the skin that diminishes naturally as we age, is collagen. Making up 75% of our skin, collagen is responsible for maintaining that thick, supple, taut appearance. As such it is such a large molecule, collagen cannot not penetrate the skin when applied to the skin in the form of a cream or serum, making peptides a great alternative. Peptides are blessed with the ability to signal cells to make more collagen and repair damaged cell structures.

Do I Look Younger Yet?!

The amount of time needed to see the results of a peptide formulated product depends largely on your skin's specific situation and type. I know its hard to read, but the key to achieving the desired results of these products is patience. Be religious about applying your products. Most of time, noticeable results will become apparent at least a month of routine application. For some, results can take up to three months. But do not let this deter you!

Remember to keep in mind that different product consistencies work differently, even if the ingredients are exactly the same. While peptide creams are beneficial for the skin, they may be too heavy. A cream's thick consistency may diminish the effectiveness of active ingredients, as they cannot fully penetrate the skin. Serums, however, allow the peptides and other active ingredients to penetrate the skin more quickly, producing more meaningful results. Try incorporating a peptide cream and serum into your daily routine to achieve more noticeable results.

Step 5:

The Fifth step nourish the upper layers of the skin and gives energy and moisture to the cells. These precious serums contain cutting-edge ingredients in the battle against time, botanical extracts with a variety of Vitamins, Peptides, Antioxidants, Hyaluronic and amino acid as well as potent moisturizing and essential oils.

The serums also stabilize the products applied during the preliminary Stages and enhance the creams that will come in the next phase. These serums prolong the effects of the skin care system. Excellent results are achieved with regular application and prevents from the skin to mature before time.

Products to us: Vitamins, Minerals, antioxidants, Serum etc

Vitamins And Anti-Oxidants

You probably already know the three surest ways to ensure youthful skin: Protect your skin from the sun, don't smoke, and eat a healthy diet. In addition, a variety of vitamins and antioxidants may also improve the health and quality of your skin.

Here are a few of the most effective ones:

1. **Vitamins C and E and Selenium for Your Skin -** Research has found that vitamins C and E, as well as selenium, can help protect the skin against sun damage and skin cancer. And they may actually reverse some of the discoloration and wrinkles associated with aging. These antioxidants work by speeding up the

skin's natural repair systems and by directly inhibiting further damage.

2. **Alpha-lipoic Acid for Your Skin -** This antioxidant, when applied topically as a cream, may help protect the skin from sun damage. Studies have looked at creams with 3%-5% concentration, applied every other day and building up slowly to once daily, and found some improvement in sun-induced changes in the skin.

3. **Coenzyme Q10 for Your Skin -** Coenzyme Q10 is a natural antioxidant in the body that helps the cells grow and protects them from the ravages of cancer. A drop in natural levels of coenzyme Q10 that occurs in our later years is thought to contribute to aging skin. A study published in the journal Biofactors found that applying coenzyme Q10 to the skin helped minimize the appearance of wrinkles.

4. **Other Antioxidants -** Many other plant-based extracts are being studied for their positive effects on the skin, either when ingested or applied topically. Examples are rosemary, tomato paste (lycopene), grape seed extract, pomegranate, and soy. Some experts feel that a blend of many different antioxidants and extracts

might be more effective than individual products. The final answer about the best doses and extracts remains to be determined by researchers.

The Important Of Serums For The Face

By now, we all know the basic skincare commandments: don't go to sleep with your makeup on. Always moisturize. Use SPF like your life depends on it. But there's a new complexion mandate you might not be as familiar with: use a serum. We're serious; adding serums to our skincare routine has made the biggest difference to the way our faces look and feel.

Not convinced? Allow us to persuade you further. Here are five big, beautiful importants of adding a serum to your skincare routine.

1. They work - Serums are all killer and no filler, containing the highest concentration of active ingredients that you can get without a prescription. Compare—cleansers and moisturizers usually contain between 5 and 10% active ingredient, whereas serums can contain up to 70%. This means that you'll actually get results, whether you're looking to even tone, reduce fine lines, brighten, firm or get rid of dark spots.

2. Zero fillers - If you have sensitive or breakout-prone skin, you know how important avoiding cheap occlusive agents (like mineral oil and petroleum) can be. Because serums are especially designed to be delivery systems, they don't contain any of those. Their goal is to make sure that their fancy active ingredients (peptides, stem cells, vitamins and beneficial minerals) get past the outer layer of your skin and deliver their greatness deep down, so anything that could get in the way of that mission is left out of the cocktail entirely. The result? A pure, potent skincare potion.

3. Fewer breakouts - People with acne-prone skin, rejoice! Unlike traditional moisturizers (which can leave a pore-blocking layer atop the skin), serums have a watery consistency — and many are, in fact, water-based instead of being oil-based. This means they absorb much faster without any breakout-encouraging residue left behind. It's the miracle we've been waiting for!

4. A less oily complexion - It happens to us on the regular: when our skin gets oily, the last thing we want to do is moisturize and add more fuel to the grease-fire. But then our sebaceous glands go bonkers, overproducing oil to try to compensate for what it feels like is chronic dryness. So our attempts to make our skin less oily actually end up making us oilier! Where will the madness end?

That's where serums come in. Far lighter (and faster to absorb) than moisturizer, they keep your skin hydrated without contributing to that greasy feeling that we all hate so much. And because you're keeping hydrated, your skin won't go nuts overproducing sebum—thus making you less oily in the long run.

5. You'll save money - But wait, we hear you saying. Serums are more expensive than any other skincare product. How will that save me money?

A Simple Tip: if you invest in a good serum, you'll actually have something that works. No more wasting money on multiple products that are just ok, or that you think might be working; a great serum is actually going to give you visible results.

It all comes down to what you'd rather spend money on: five cheaper products that take up space on your shelf and do nothing for your skin, or one product that does amazing things and costs a little more. Trust us: once you find your perfect serum, you'll never waste your dollars on anything else again.

Step 6:

The creams and masks are the Sixth stage and are applied to the face, neck and cleavage. They contribute balanced botanical, biological and Nano Tech elements to the skin. They supplement the actions of the Nurture serums and protect the skin from dryness. The creams are easy to apply and are rich in active ingredients providing optimum results with a nut-sized amount. Most Beauty programs include two different hydrating creams, one for day time and one for night time.

Products to use: Emollients, hydrants, butters, oils

Importance Of Hydrating The Skin

The Importance of hydrating the skin from a young age to defy the signs of time and help the skin moist itself. People with dry, itchy, aging skin often do not drink enough water to keep the skin healthy and soft. One of the most important things you can do for your skin's health and appearance is to stay hydrated. Your skin is made up of three main layers consist of seven layers: the outer layer (epidermis), the underlying skin (dermis), and the subcutaneous tissue. When the outermost layer of your skin does not contain enough moisture, the skin will lose its elasticity and feel rough.

Staying hydrated will rejuvenate your skin so it looks and feels smooth and soft. This is due to the fact that the outermost layer of the skin has the moisture it needs to flush away toxins and carry nutrients to the skin's cells. Skin that is well-hydrated also is less sensitive to irritants and germs that can slip through the lipid barrier when the skin lacks moisture.

Skin that is lacking the hydration it needs often becomes itchy, flaky, red, or even inflamed. Dry skin can even exaggerate the appearance of fine lines and wrinkles due to shrinkage of skin cells.

Why Is It Important To Keep The Skin Hydrated?

When skin is well-hydrated, it is more plump and resilient. This is due, at least in part, to an ingredient in the skin called hyaluronic acid. The job of hyaluronic acid in the skin is to hold water. When there is adequate water from inside and out the skin looks healthier and more vibrant and is less prone to wrinkles. It is important to drink lots of fluids throughout the day for best results. You've probably heard that drinking six to eight glasses of water a day is a good idea but you may need more or less depending on your activity level. Coffee and sodas do not count as water because they contain caffeine which is a diuretic, meaning that they draw water out of your system and your skin.

In order for the skin to protect our bodies from UV radiation, microorganisms and toxic agents, it must be kept adequately hydrated. Hydrated skin will remain flexible and allow our protective barrier to remain intact. If skin is broken, environmental factors can damage our bodies and cause exacerbated water loss, feeding a cyclical pattern of more damage due to further dehydration.

Moisturizing Daily For Soft, Supple Skin

Skin professionals recommend using a moisturizer daily. Moisturizers should include ingredients in one of three different classes to help promote skin hydration:

1. Humectant

2. Emollient

3. Occlusive

1. **Humectant -** Humectants are ingredients that bind water to the stratum corneum (the outermost layer of the skin). These ingredients draw moisture from the environment, but also carry it from the deeper layers of the skin to the surface. Sodium PCA, butylene glycol, glycerin, and hyaluronic acid are all examples of humectants.

2. **Emollient -** Emollients provide skin with a soft, pliable feel. This class of ingredients remains on the skin's surface, lubricating, reducing flakiness, and improving the overall appearance. Examples of emollients include lipids and oils. Shea butter, algae extract, and phosphatidylcholine are examples of emollients.

3. **Occlusive -** Occlusive ingredients help hold water in the skin by slowing down evaporation. Similar to emollients, these products remain on the surface, creating a thin film that helps block the loss of water. While historically this was thought to cause

comedones — whiteheads and blackheads — these ingredients do not necessarily clog pores or create issues for the skin. Silicones, like dimethicone and cyclomethicone, are commonly used occlusives in personal care products. These ingredients work together to restore the balance between TEWL and skin hydration. When skin is well-hydrated, it is more plump and resilient. This is due, at least in part, to an ingredient in the skin called hyaluronic acid. The job of hyaluronic acid in the skin is to hold water. When there is adequate water from inside and out the skin looks healthier and more vibrant and is less prone to wrinkles. It is important to drink lots of fluids throughout the day for best results. You've probably heard that drinking six to eight glasses of water a day is a good idea but you may need more or less depending on your activity level. Coffee and sodas do not count as water because they contain caffeine which is a diuretic, meaning that they draw water out of your system and your skin.

Step 7:

Protective products are the Seventh step and are used for the finishing touches. These products are the last and most important treatment during the day. We strongly recommend using the protection products in the morning and to repeat applying them a few more times during the day. Using them over the creams gives the skin a natural durable protection.

Products to use: sun screens, BB creams, powders and make up

Make Up And Sun Screens

Make up as a sun screen protector but never without sun screen underneath

Although dermatologists recommend wearing sunscreen every day, most people don't. Unless your foundation has an SPF already in the formula, it's recommended that you apply some sort of SPF face lotion before applying any face makeup. Some dermatologists even recommend wearing sunscreen even if your foundation has an SPF in it.

Most drug stores and beauty stores have sunscreens to match all of your skin-type needs, from oily to dry skin. Choose one that you like so that it becomes habitual; when temperature does start to heat up, you won't forget to apply your sunscreen every morning. SPF should be 15 or higher and be reapplied every two hours. The SPF value indicates the level of sunburn protection provided by the sunscreen product.

" The [SPF] test measures the amount of ultraviolet (UV) radiation exposure it takes to cause sunburn when a person is using a sunscreen in comparison to how much UV exposure it takes to cause a sunburn when they do not use a sunscreen," says the FDA.

If you're going to be outdoors in the sun or even it's cloudy, you definitely need sunscreen. Even when you have makeup on, a little touch-up of your sun block is recommended, especially if you're going to be in the sun. There are powder formulas available so that your cream foundation won't smear, run, or rub off. Sunscreens with broad spectrum protection (against UVA and UVB rays) and with sun protection factor (SPF) values of 30 or higher are recommended. The SPF number is the level of protection the sunscreen provides against UVB rays - a higher number means more protection

Many people, especially younger men and women, don't realize the skin-damaging effects the sun can have. The ugly head of sun damage doesn't rear its head till people are much older and by then the effects can't be reversed and can lead to more than just prematurely aged skin it can lead to skin cancer.

Make sure that you let your sunscreen dry before you put on any makeup or any other creams. Also, be aware of the directions of how to apply it. Most bottles recommend applying liberally and applying it all over your face, ears, neck and arms.

Being aware of putting sunscreen on every is going to help your skin in the long run, but if you skip a day here and there especially when you're not in the direct sun it won't cause any detrimental effects. "If you're just going from your car to your office or you're going to be outside for small periods of time then it's not necessary to always wear sunscreen under your makeup.

Sun Damage And The Importance
Of Sun Screen And BB Cream

Although most people love the warmth and light of the sun, too much sun exposure can significantly damage human skin. The sun's heat dries out areas of unprotected skin and depletes the skin's supply of natural lubricating oils. In addition, the sun's ultraviolet (UV) radiation can cause burning and long-term changes in the skin's structure.

The most common types of sun damage to the skin are:

1. **Dry skin** — Sun-exposed skin can gradually lose moisture and essential oils, making it appear dry, flaky and prematurely wrinkled, even in younger people.

2. **Sunburn** — Sunburn is the common name for the skin injury that appears immediately after the skin is exposed to UV radiation. Mild sunburn causes only painful reddening of the skin, but more severe cases can produce tiny fluid-filled bumps (vesicles) or larger blisters.

3. **Actinic keratosis** — This is a tiny bump that feels like sandpaper or a small, scaly patch of sun-damaged skin

that has a pink, red, yellow or brownish tint. Unlike suntan markings or sunburns, an actinic keratosis does not usually go away unless it is frozen, chemically treated or removed by a doctor. An actinic keratosis develops in areas of skin that have undergone repeated or long-term exposure to the sun's UV light, and it is a warning sign of increased risk of skin cancer. About 10% to 15% of actinic keratoses eventually change into squamous cell cancers of the skin.

4. **Long-term changes in the skin's collagen (a structural protein)** — These changes include photoaging (premature aging of the skin because of sun exposure) and actinic purpura (bleeding from fragile blood vessels beneath the skin surface). In photoaging, the skin develops wrinkles and fine lines because of changes in the collagen of a deep layer of the skin called the dermis. In actinic purpura, UV radiation damages the structural collagen that supports the walls of the skin's tiny blood vessels. Particularly in older people, this collagen damage makes blood vessels more fragile and more likely to rupture following a slight impact.

Over a lifetime, repeated episodes of sunburn and unprotected sun exposure can increase a person's risk of malignant melanoma and other forms of skin cancer. As a rule, if you have fair skin and light eyes, you are at greater risk of sun-related skin damage and skin cancers. This is because your skin contains less of a dark pigment called melanin, which helps to protect the skin from the effects of UV radiation.

The painful redness of sunburn will fade within a few days, provided that you do not re-expose your injured skin to the sun without using a sunblock or sunscreen. Some sun damage is permanent, although prescription medications, nonprescription remedies and skin-resurfacing treatments may improve the skin's appearance.

Prevention

You can help to prevent sun-damaged skin by taking the following steps:

1. Apply a sunscreen before you go outdoors

Choose a water-resistant sunscreen that has a sun protection factor (SPF) of 30 or above, with a broad spectrum of protection against both UV-A and UV-B rays. Be sure to reapply often to avoid sweating off or washing off the sunscreen.

What are the top five reasons you believe everyone should wear sunscreen?

- The ozone layer is depleting and your body needs shielding from harmful rays.

- Skin cancer rates are on the rise and sunscreen has been proven to decrease the development of skin cancer.

- It helps to prevent facial brown spots and skin discolorations.

- It also helps to reduce the appearance of facial red veins and blotchiness.

- It slows down the development of wrinkled, premature aging skin.

2. Use a BB cream that can work to reflect the rays of the sun

What are BB cream?

You may have heard the name BB thrown around but what exactly is it? BB creams are 'beauty balms' or 'blemish balms'. These are designed to provide the skin with a light coverage while also moisturising, reflecting light and offering SPF protection! But I wouldn't trust them to be my only protection against the sun always use them after a sun block of at least 30 SPF.

Night Time Tip to Remember – At Night when you are not using a sun screen, use a rich face balm or a night mask that is good to use without washing. This will insure the work off all layers that were applied before.

Chapter 6

Your Skin Care Regime

One of the top questions we're asked on the regular is actually pretty basic: "What should my skin-care routine look like?"

it can be incredibly daunting to figure out exactly what you should be doing to your face. Then there's the question of what order it should be done and how, exactly, should common products be applied? Don't fret, because we're here to give you a beauty road map that answers all of these questions and more. Ahead, you'll find a basic skin-care routine anyone can follow, no matter your skin type. It lays out the basics: makeup remover, cleanser, serum, moisturizer, and sunscreen.

How many layers to use

The number of layers recommended; is your age divided to 10, for example: in your 30's you need 3 layers, in your 40's you need 4 layers and so on.

If you are only beginning to treat your skin with Professional products and you feel you want to start with less layers to get accustomed to the process, it is good as well. With Time you will be acquainted with the products and their benefits and you will be able to use more layers to get better results. With this we recommend, for the long run, not to compromise and use all needed layers in order to provide the skin all active and nourishing substances and enjoy the amazing results of using it.

Changes Throughout The Ages

Want to know what's happened to your skin and what the future holds? The below decade-by-decade guide will give you the information you need to understand changes past, present, and future. In the next section, we will also identify and detail the appropriate skincare routine that best meets the demands of these changes, at each stage, to keep your skin looking its best!

In our 20s, our skin is besieged by free radical damage (from our hectic schedules, sun-worshiping, pollution, and so much more). Free radicals are atoms, molecules, or ions that can cause cell damage and death. Our newly independent lifestyles (complete with more stress and less sleep) can lead to a "toxin overload" that shows up on our faces through bags, puffiness, and dullness. Among other health issues, free radicals can accelerate the aging of our skin. Antioxidants, like vitamin A, vitamin C, and vitamin E, fight free radical damage. As a result, twenty-something women need antioxidants in their skincare products to repair skin and protect it against future damage and premature wrinkles. In her 20s, one of the most important anti-aging steps a woman can take is to wear sunscreen every day.

Sunscreen is necessary no matter what your age, but the younger a woman starts a daily SPF regimen, the better off her skin will be in the future. Although the face is typically the biggest area of concern for future wrinkles, it is critical to protect all exposed skin, including the neck, chest, hands, and legs. Sun damage in the 20s can also lead to discoloration in the form of sun spots. Protecting skin with a high SPF, exfoliating regularly, and delivering antioxidants are keys to successful skincare for the 20s.

In our 30s, most women begin to see their first fine lines and wrinkles. Simultaneously, their levels of collagen and elastin decrease and skin tone becomes duller and more uneven.

Skin regeneration now takes twice as long, leading to a loss in elasticity, uneven tone, and new wrinkles, particularly around the eyes. Discoloration is also starting to emerge, typically as a result of sun damage or melasma. The thirty-something woman requires ingredients in her skincare products that address all of these issues!

As in her 20s, she needs products that deliver antioxidants to the skin to reverse the damage caused by free radicals and protect it from future damage. Natural exfoliants are also critical in her skincare products to help offset skin's slowed regeneration rate. Products with retinoid ingredients can help even out her skin tone. Finally, a slightly thicker moisturizer with hyaluronic acid can help restore the hydration and suppleness of her skin and reduce the appearance of her new fine lines and wrinkles.

In our 40s, we face a new foe: thinning skin. Thinner skin leads to dryer skin, a drop in elasticity, and duller tone. A drop in elasticity means that wrinkles become deeper and lines of movement between the brows and around the eyes and mouth don't disappear completely like they used to. Simultaneously in our 40s, skin sensitivity increases, as demonstrated by more freckles, sun spots, and spider veins.

Skin in its 40s requires specific ingredients to improve elasticity, tone, hydration, and firmness as well as ingredients to target signs of photo-aging and sun sensitivity. Peptides can help to stimulate collagen and elastin production for firmer, tighter skin. A thicker cream with hyaluronic acid can also help increased the skin's moisturization for improved elasticity, smoother tone, and reduced appearance of wrinkles.

In our 50s and beyond, hormonal changes threaten to send skin- aging into overdrive. Our skin experiences a rapid decline in surface immunity while the natural moisture barrier further degrades, leading to even thinner and drier skin. Moreover, wrinkles gain definition, pores become larger, and age spots begin to appear. Skincare ingredients must be hydrating, firming, and reinforcing to battle these effects of our bodies' changing hormones! Plenty of moisture and hydration is needed to maintain your healthy glow at this stage. Effective ingredients including peptides, hyaluronic acid, retinoids, and key amino acids are critical to anti-wrinkle and general anti-aging skincare success in the 50s. Powerful antioxidants, like resveratrol, can help target new imperfections and discolorations. Skin creams should be thick and hydrating to restore the suppleness and glowing tone to your skin. Frequent exfoliation can also help to encourage cell regeneration for tighter, firmer skin.

Routines That Fit Each Stage

Energizing Skincare Regimen for your 20s!

Cleanse! Use a gentle foaming cleanser to rid skin of those damaging free radicals every morning and every night before you go to bed. Choose a cleanser that can effectively remove makeup residue and excess oil to avoid clogged pores and unwanted bacteria.

Moisturize daily! Use a light, non-greasy moisturizer that provides UVA and UVB protection. Moisturizers should list zinc oxide, titanium dioxide, avobenzone or mexoryl to indicate ingredients that protect you against the sun. If your moisturizer does not list any of these ingredients, be sure to layer an SPF product on top of it daily, before any sun exposure.

Extra Tips: It is especially critical to cleanse your face well at night if you have been exposed to smoke and pollution during the day. Post-cleansing, applying a cream or lotion with vitamin C can help offset some of the damage that exposure to these toxins can cause.

Refreshing Skincare Regimen for your 30s!

Cleanse! It's time to switch over to a non-foaming cleanser that won't dry out your skin. Follow up every facial cleansing with a hydrating moisturizer. Make sure you're drinking plenty of water throughout the day as well to ensure hydration from the inside and out!

Moisturize daily! To reduce damage caused from sun (both today and in years past) use a moisturizer that has powerful antioxidants layered with an SPF product. This helps guard against more damage and even reverse damage from those times you tried the tanning bed or sat outside covered in baby oil! Botanicals, seaweed and fruit extracts are great ingredients to have in your products as well. Not only are they naturally based, but they also help the skin restore its own exfoliation and regeneration capacities by stimulating the activity of skin enzymes in the natural process of regeneration. Some can also help reduce oxidative skin stressor molecules and most have soothing and calming effects on the skin.

Extra Tips: Don't over-treat your skin in your 30s. If you feel you need a stronger skincare product, choose one that is higher in vitamin A or retinoids (which are chemically related). Both ingredients promote better skin tone and texture.

Invigorating Skincare Regimen for your 40s!

Cleanse and Exfoliate! It is important to gently scrub and wash away dead skin cells to keep your skin looking healthy. As in your 30s, choose a basic non-foaming cleanser that also adds hydration back to your skin. The skin of a woman in her 40s tends to be drier, so it is important to avoid stripping away natural oils with a harsh cleanser. Look for ingredients like aloe and chamomile that help retain moisture and are soothing on skin; avoid soaps and cleansers that are acidic. Finally, choose a thick, hydrating scrub to exfoliate your skin on a weekly basis. Follow up every exfoliation and cleansing by applying a hydrating moisturizer.

Moisturize Daily! As at every age, you should protect yourself from sun damage every day with an SPF! To help with the damage you may already have, choose skincare products that are high in powerful antioxidants. Grapeseed extract and resveratrol are great examples of natural and powerful antioxidants. Resveratrol is a botanical compound and powerful antioxidant found in the skin of red grapes. Many studies on this polyphenol have indicated its potential as an anti-aging, anti-inflammatory, and UVB protection active. It can protect collagen to help offset declines in skin elasticity. In our 40s, it is also important to use a night cream to help our skin retain as much moisture as possible. Choose a moisturizing night cream that includes glycerin or hyaluronic acid to help your skin retain the moisture it needs for a youthful glow. Using a night cream is also important at this time to retain as much moisture as possible. Use a moisturizer that includes glycerin or hyaluronic acid to help your skin retain the moisture it needs for that youthful glow.

Extra Tips! Peptides are becoming proven warriors in the fight against signs of aging. They can help boost and reactivate the collagen your skin is losing. For example, tetrapeptide-17 is an anti-aging peptide that helps stimulate collagen and elastin production. It has a unique peptide sequence based on the skin's own structure and has shown potential to counterbalance the degradation of the extra-cellular matrix (ECM) of the skin as well as its ability to stimulate collagen synthesis.

Rejuvenating Skincare Regimen for your 50s!

Cleanse! Now is the time to choose a cream cleanser that will add hydration back to your skin while it cleanses away the impurities of the day. In your 50s+, hydration is the key to youthful, supple skin. The use of a cream- based, exfoliating scrub with natural ingredients will also help improve skin texture and tone by gently removing dead skin cells. Follow up every exfoliation and cleansing by generously applying a thick, hydrating moisturizer.

Moisturize Daily! Our skin's sensitivity has increased by the time we reach our 50s so use caution when selecting a moisturizer. Look for one that is fragrance-free and has been formulated for sensitive skin. Also, select a cream that contains hyaluronic acid. Hyaluronic acid has been shown to significantly improve skin elasticity, reduce skin roughness, and reduce the appearance of wrinkles. Creamy moisturizers that are high in hyaluronic acid can also help your thirsty skin improve its moisture barrier so it can retain moisture better.

Extra Tips! Many women in their 50s+ choose to add a hydrating serum to their skincare routine. Serums typically are used to get added nutrients into deeper layers of the skin that a regular moisturizer cannot reach as effectively. Choose a serum that is high in anti- aging ingredients (especially peptides and hyaluronic acid) and apply it after your moisturizing cream to seal in hydration even more.

CONCLUSION

From our 20s until way beyond our 60s, we are inundated with promises, products, and services that guarantee younger- looking skin. Whether they come from new surgeries, expensive injections, diets, creams, serums, lasers, or so something else, it's very hard to tell what will work and what's a waste of time, money, and energy! We understand and we hope this book has helped you to learn more about your skin, how it's changing, and what you can do daily to keep it as young and beautiful as possible.

With the layer system Results are accumulating over time. Roller help to penetrating ingredients to the skin and multiply the efficiency of products, The best way to maximize the efficiency of skin care are professional creams. The Layer system is at home procedure with best known results. The best way to treat the skin is with professional and natural products.

It's never too late to start taking the best care of your skin. Looking great is hard work, but it can be fun too. Best of all, the results make it all worthwhile! Now that you're armed with the information to improve your skin and protect against future aging, you're ready to become one of those women who looks better and better with age!

In the end, ageing is a natural process. No amount of age-defying or anti-wrinkle cream or gels, injections or liposuction can stop the inevitable designed by Mother Nature. Women who accept this will live happier.

Thank you very much for reading the book. If you loved the book, I would appreciate it if you can write a review of the book for me. If you have any question about the book feel free to contact me at orilaor@outlook.com.

For 20$ Coupon for www.laorcare.com were you can find all the professional products to clear your Pigmentation, send the word: BEAUTIFUL to my mail.

With sincere love Ori Laor